ABOUT this BOOK

This book is a bit of a departure for me in that it is obviously *not* a children's book. It has exactly the same format as the *Fran's Van* children's books but is a road trip for very different travellers. Although the menopause is referred to, it is not the only thing which was on my mind as I wrote this book. Having got a little bit older I have become aware of what it is to become a grey-haired 'elder' woman. There is little change to how I feel on the inside and how much I want to get out of life, but huge changes to how I look. It seems that as we age, society judges the external and loses interest in the person behind the fading pigment and the stiffening joints. Many of the women I taught with over the years talked about becoming increasingly invisible as they got older. This is a story about women who are refusing to be invisible, and also about the sisterhood of the shared experience of the menopause and the ageing process.

The menopause affects us in different ways and at different ages, but talking about it, understanding it and sharing experiences means that we can understand that we are not alone – especially as it can last for up to fifteen years. The menopause can give women black days, sleepless nights, mood swings and temperature changes which can stop you thinking. So to all of you out there, whether you are living it, remembering it, or looking forward to it, bring it on as we are up to the job.

Enjoy this foray into the sisterhood and remember: age is just a number.

£2.45

To Ishbel
with best wishes
Fran

Fran's Van
and the
Four Menopausal Women

Frances Herbert

Published by Frances Herbert
Publishing partner: Paragon Publishing, Rothersthorpe
First published 2017

All characters and stories created by Frances Herbert
Illustrations by Frances Herbert

ISBN 978-1-78222-561-4

Book design, layout and production management by Into Print
www.intoprint.net
01604 832149

Printed and bound in UK and USA by Lightning Source

ECO Credentials
Lightning Source has received Chain of Custody (CoC) certification from:
The Sustainable Forestry Initiative® (SFI®).
The Forest Stewardship Council™ (FSC®)
Programme for the Endorsement of Forest Certification™ (PEFC™)

Chain of Custody (CoC) is an accounting system that tracks wood fiber through the different stages of production: from the forest, to the mill, to the paper, to the printer and ultimately to the finished book.
For further detailed information please visit:

http://lightningsource.com/ChainOfCustody/

Thanks to:

Jackie Ross for encouraging me to publish this book, and to all my fantastic women friends who have been there at every stage of my life.

It was five weeks since Fran had moved into her new house and she had still to unpack the last few boxes. Opening a bottle of wine and summoning up the energy to tackle at least one more box she dragged a cardboard carton marked “kitchen” to the front of the fire and started to work her way through. It was full of ornaments, small pictures and at the bottom, her hand felt a round, flat disc. Dragging it out of the box she held it in front of the fire and recognised the small stained glass disc which depicted her old camper van – Dora. Fran held it up to the fire, the dancing flames lit up the colours of the glass and suddenly Fran’s head was filled with memories of all the adventures she had had with Dora and her children. They had rescued, among other things, an otter, a naughty dog, and a puffer owner. They had driven all over the west of Scotland and they had met many interesting characters.

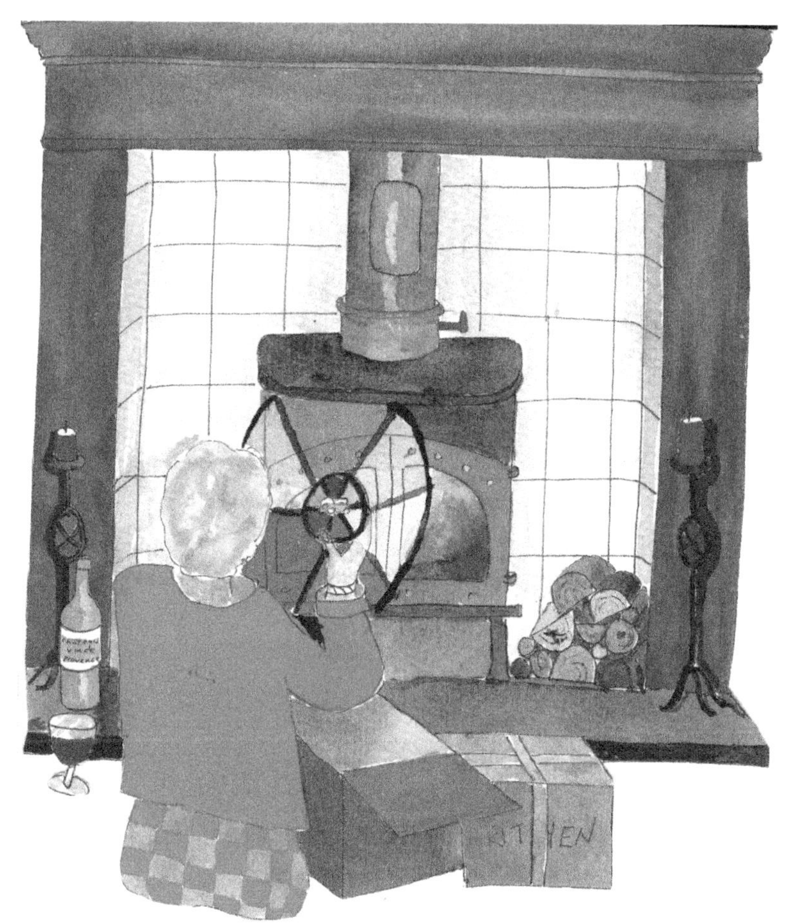

She sat back on her haunches and felt a great sadness when she thought of her children now all grown up and gone from home. Images of the west of Scotland where they had taken so many happy holidays in their ancient Volkswagen camper van – Pandora, or Dora for short – flew into her head.

Fran still owned Dora, how could she ever have sold her? That being said she had left her languishing in the garage as Dora was now forty-three years old and needed a great deal of work done to make her road worthy. Friends had laughed when she had insisted on taking Dora when she moved but she could not have left her.

On their final journey together Dora's wiring loom had developed a fault and melted. Since that undignified return home on the back of a breakdown lorry, Dora had not been on the road.

Fran had a sudden need to see Dora. She picked up her glass of wine, pulled on her shoes and made her way to Dora's garage. Dragging the door open she stared down at her beloved van and felt a sudden wave of nostalgia so strong that it caught in her throat and brought tears to her eyes. Fran took a long drink of her wine and put her hand onto Dora's windscreen.

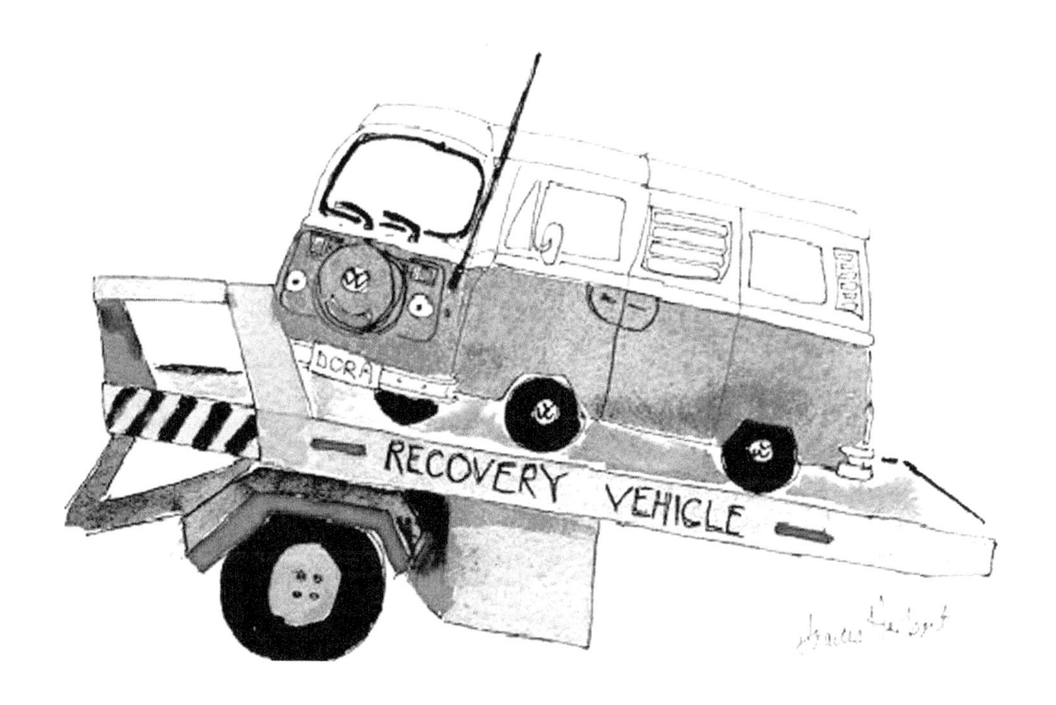

Dora sat there, solid on her old tires, her paintwork dull and covered in dirt. Fran felt guilty but also the stirrings of an idea.

> *"Sleep well Dora, I am thinking we have one more great adventure left in us."* Fran gently shut the door.

*

It took several months for Dora to become road worthy. She needed new tyres, a new exhaust and, of course, a complete new wiring loom. There was some rust to deal with and a great deal of cleaning and polishing but finally Fran decided that Dora was ready for the road.

Fran thought long and hard about what to do on her adventure but could find no inspiration. She knew exactly who she would invite on her trip – her three best friends from school – Helen, Betty, and Joni – but what was she going to say to them, what could she offer to entice them to travel in an ancient van with very simple facilities? They would be cramped and uncomfortable and none of them was in the first flush of youth. How should she play this?

Finishing off a final polish on Dora's front panel, she explained her dilemma to Dora.

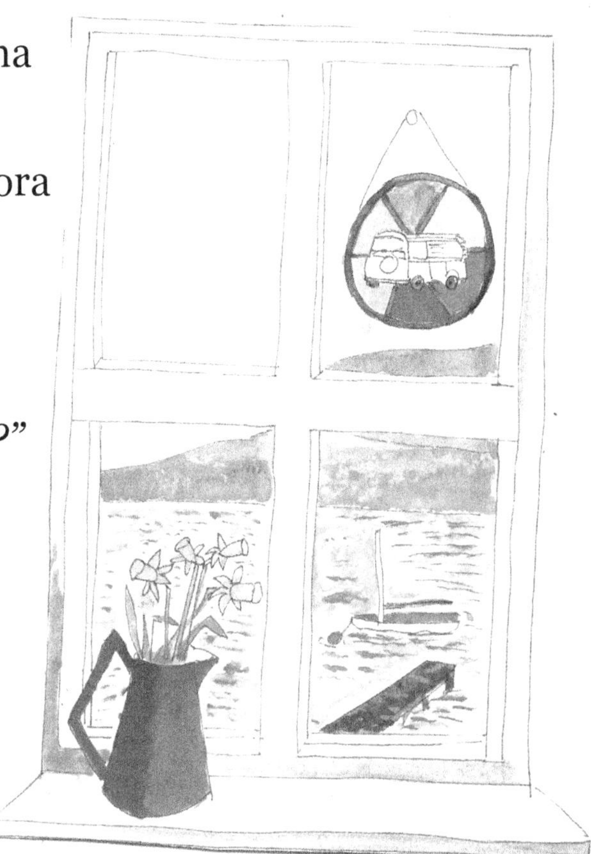

"Well it's obvious isn't it?" stated Dora in her condescending manner.

"Well no, not to me."

"Have you hung up the stained glass window in your new kitchen?"

"No, I never thought to, do you think the magic is still there after all these years?"

"There is always magic if you are open to it," Dora said, *"the magic must still be there. For heavens sake, you are having a conversation with a VW campervan. What do you think?"*

Fran dropped her polishing rag and ran to find the colourful disc. Sticking it to the window, she looked over her shoulder but there was no reflection on the kitchen wall.

Fran sighed but feeling more positive and that her hair-brained scheme had at least a starting point, she decided to write invitations which would encourage her friends to join her.

Sitting back she admired the handiwork of her handmade card. She hadn't actually told them where they were going but then, she couldn't. She hadn't told them when they were going but then, she couldn't.

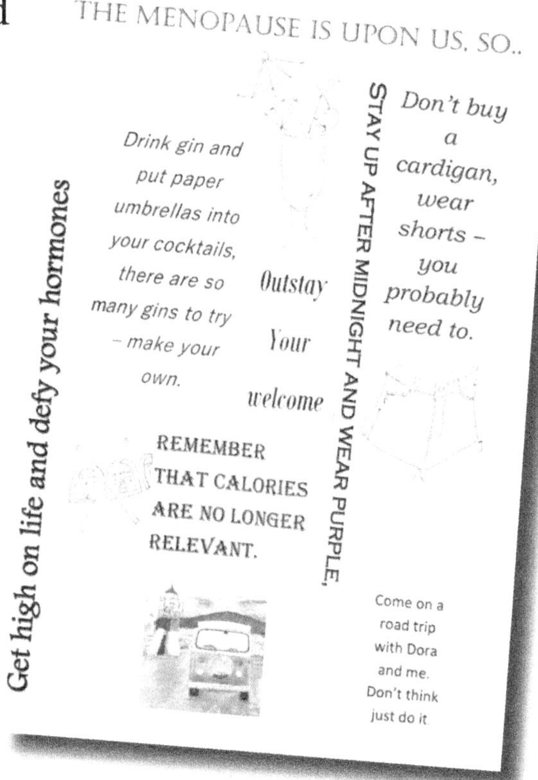

Sitting back in her chair she felt the undeniable flush of heat which seemed to start at her feet and radiate through her whole body. What was she thinking?

Betty phoned first.

"Hi, Fran?" Betty always sounded surprised when she used a mobile phone that it actually worked and that she had actually managed to reach the person she had phoned.

"Yes, it's me. Hi, Betty!"

"How did you know it was me?"

"Voice recognition you know." Fran sighed. It was always the same with Betty. *"You got my invitation?"*

"Is that what it was, an invitation. I thought it was one of your art thingies."

"Ah, right, anyway what do you think? Are you up for it?"

"Well, when are we going and where are we going and are you seriously thinking that we should go in that old van of yours? I assume you've invited the others. That means there will be four of us in that old van."

Fran took a deep breath, why had she not thought this through? *"I can't tell you that yet?"*

"What, you can't tell me anything?"

"Well, I can, we're going in Dora and yes, I've invited the others and that "old van" has been well and truly fettled and is raring to go. She's more than up to the job."

There was a silence from Betty.

"Where are we going to sleep?"

"In Dora, of course." Fran tried to sound upbeat.

"What! Good grief. Surely that's going to be really inadequate."

"Betty, you are literally sucking the life out of me. I was planning an adventure, a spontaneous event, not a trip out with the local Derby and Joan club."

There was silence from Betty.

"Let me think about it, ok. It has come out of left field a bit, you know."

There was silence from Betty and Fran realised she had hung up.

"Hello, is that you, Fran?"

"Yeh, hiya Helen, how are you? Did you get my invitation?"

"Yes, I did, interesting, where are we going?"

Fran felt cheered by this positive response. *"Don't know yet,"* she said.

"Sounds a bit out there. Are we really traveling in Dora, can't believe she's not gone to the big garage in the sky."

"Well, I've fettled her up within an inch of her life and she is raring to go." Fran pictured her beautiful van resting in her garage and felt relieved that Dora could not hear what was being said about her.

"Well, we will be stopping at hotels anyway surely?"

"Well no, I was thinking we would sleep in Dora."

There was a silence from Helen.

"You still there?" asked Fran.

"Yes, I'm just thinking it through. I mean Dora's not exactly well equipped is she? No shower, toilet etc...are you serious?"

"Very serious, Helen, we are talking about an adventure here, spontaneity and well..." Fran was starting to feel as if she was repeating herself.

"Ok, I will if you can at least fix a porta potty. I mean things aren't just all where they should be down below and I don't want to get caught short."

"Thanks for that, but, ok, I'll find a way of doing that. If I can are you in?"

There was a silence from Helen and then: *"Yes, good grief, we're not dead yet are we?"*

“Hello, is that you Fran?”

“Hi, Joni, yes how are you?”

“I’ve been talking to Betty and Helen and I’ve had your invite but I can’t come.”

Fran felt as if she had been kicked in the stomach. *“What, that’s it no discussion, no questions just no?”*

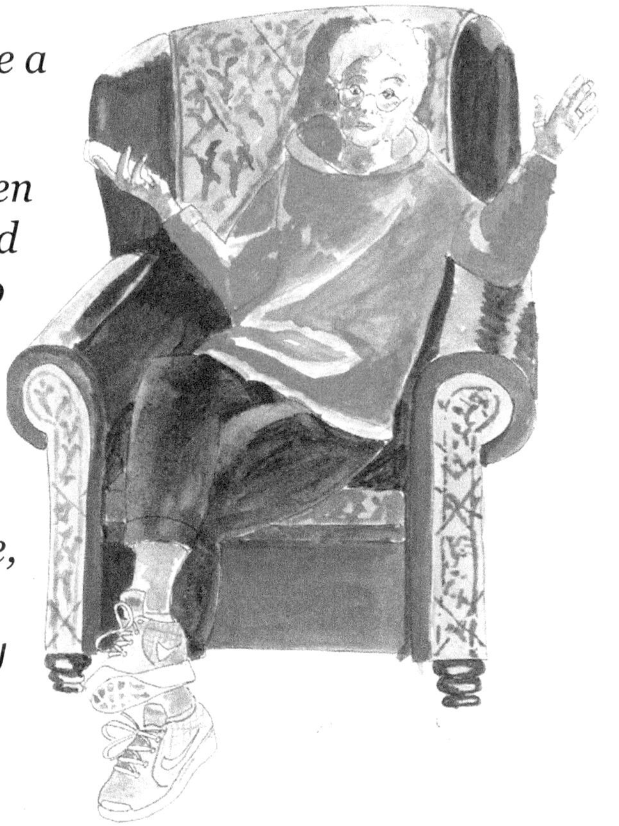

“I’m waiting to go into hospital to have a hip replacement.”

“Ah, right I see. Well, I don’t know when we’re going and so you might have had it and it could be just what you need to set you on the road to recovery.”

There was a silence from Joni. Then: *“You’re mad.”*

“Not mad, just… wanting to live a little, to forget about all the bits that hurt and go out and have some fun with my old buddies.”

"Right well, l need more information, I'll have to have a think. Get back to you soon, bye."

Feeling really deflated, Fran walked out to see Dora. She opened the door and climbed in resting her hands on Dora's steering wheel.

"When we off?" asked Dora.

"I'm not sure Dora, just not sure. I've still got a few things to sort out before we can go." Fran had had an idea.

Three days later Fran drove Dora out of her garage onto the drive. Dora was aware of some activity behind her.

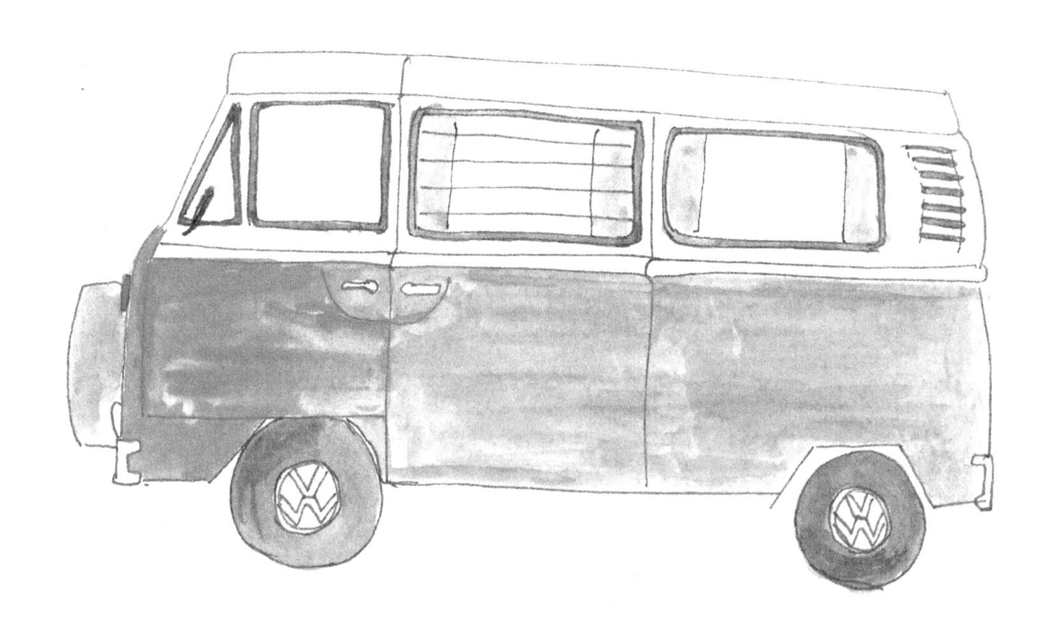

"What you doing Fran?"

"Just making some preparations for our trip. Have a look in your rearview mirror."

There was a silence from Dora.

"You are joking!" she shouted. *"Good grief, no dignity left at all."*

*

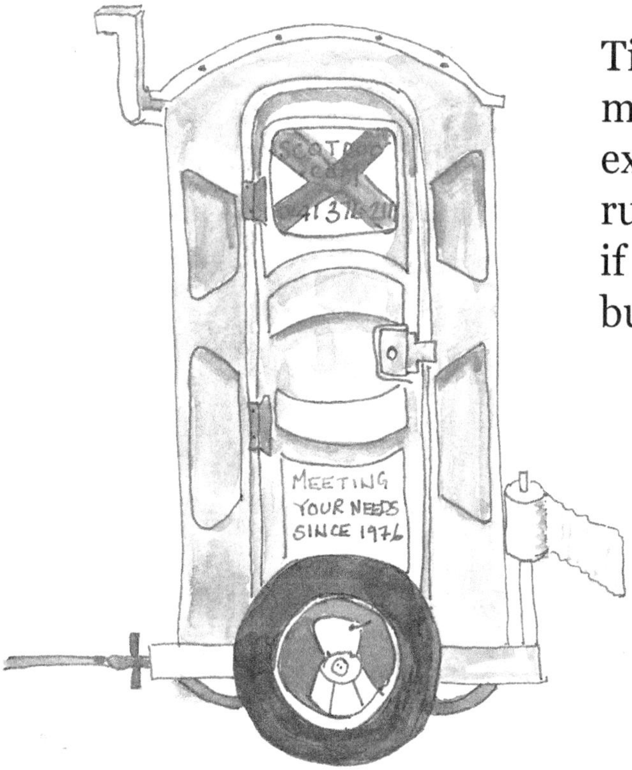

Time seemed to pass so slowly. Every morning Fran entered the kitchen with expectation, much as she did when she rushed out on spring mornings to see if her potatoes had come through, but – nothing.

The stained glass disc resolutely refused to shine and gradually other things began to take up Fran's time and energy in her newly found retirement. She took up painting with a vengeance and joined an art class. This gave her great joy but she was increasingly feeling that her life was getting smaller and she painted acrylics of the places she wanted to visit in her beloved west of Scotland.

Get a grip she told herself. You've always been the queen of nostalgia, stop being so pathetic. Make your preparations, be ready. Somewhere in the back of her mind, she knew it would all come together. She composed a text to send to her potential travel buddies:

I have no further travel information for you yet, ladies, however, please can you pack and be ready to go because when the light shines through the stained glass window you have to go with whatever you are standing in and you have only one hour before Dora and I turn up at your door. Your baggage allowance is one cabin bag. Don't worry about anything else. Be in touch soon. F

Having sent the text, Fran sat back holding her phone waiting for replies.

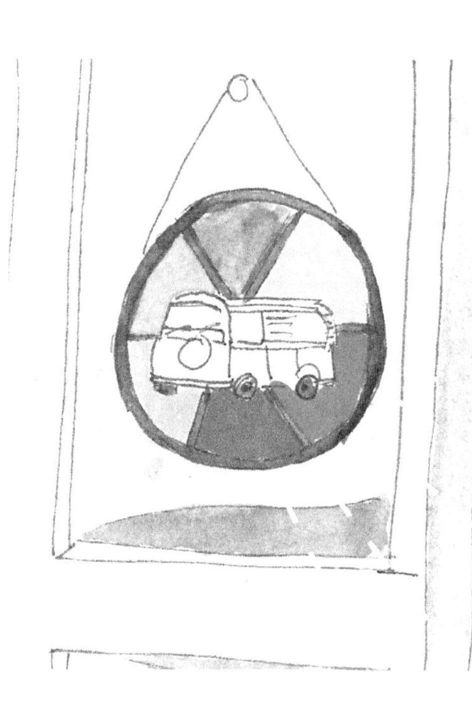

Helen first: **Good grief!**
Betty next: **Jings, crivens, help ma Bob!**
And finally Joni: **!!!!!!!!**

Right, thought Fran – we're on.

But still, the light did not shine and so Fran packed and then started to make adaptions to Dora, thinking about what four women of a certain age, traveling together, would need and what would make the trip a success.

Spring was early, the lengthening days and earlier mornings lifted Fran's spirits. Surely it wouldn't be long now. Finally one morning Fran felt a compulsion to get up very early. Light was sneaking through her bedroom curtains as she reached for her slippers.
Dressing quickly, she didn't want to raise her hopes too high but yes, finally, the day was here. The stained glass window of Dora shone a perfect reflection onto the kitchen wall. She sent a text to her unsuspecting travel companions. Grabbing her cabin bag she made her holiday safety checks, locked the house and headed for Dora's garage.

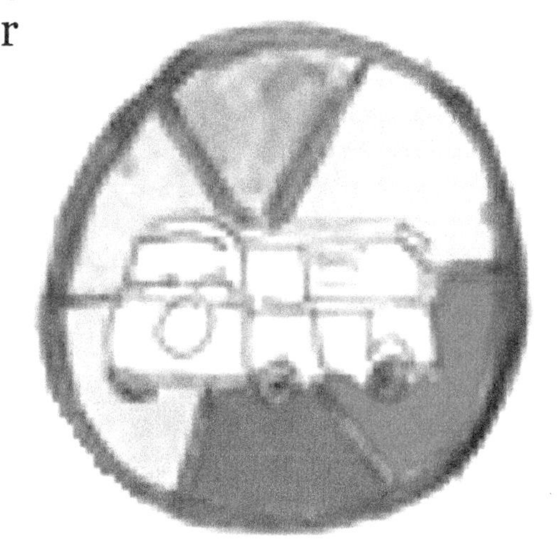

Dora looked up and seemed to stretch on her chassis. *"This the day then?"* she asked.

"Yes Dora, this is the day. Just going to look and see if the magic box has arrived." Fran slid open Dora's heavy side panel and there it was but it was not glowing. Fran tried to open the lid but it appeared to be stuck. She thought about this for a minute and then connected the trailer and set off to her first pick-up.
Fran almost ran up the house steps, raised her hand to knock, before she could, the door flew open to reveal Betty. She was dressed completely in khaki, an outrageous safari suit with a crimson and navy scarf wrapped jauntily around her neck and, to top it off, a crimson deerstalker with the flaps down. Fran's hand flew to her mouth.

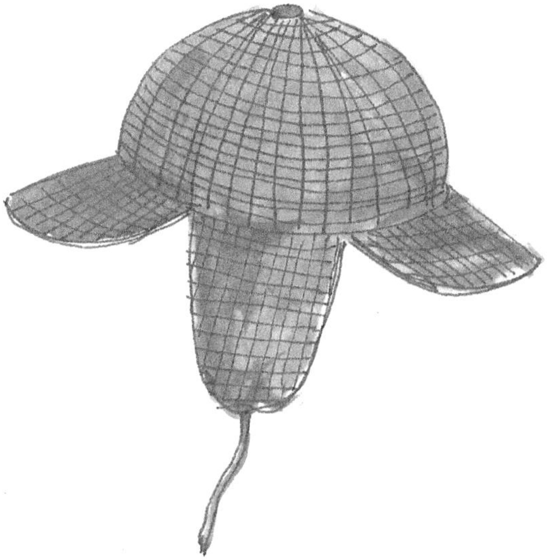

"Good grief!" Fran spluttered and then burst out laughing.

Betty contrived to look hurt and then took off the deerstalker and stated haughtily: *"Well, you said be ready and that we're going on an adventure so here I am,"* she posed, *"ready for anything."*

Fran felt suddenly really happy, it was going to be alright. Before reaching for the door to shut it behind her, Betty took off the deerstalker and threw it recklessly over her shoulder. *"Well, I don't want to look totally ridiculous."* She paused. *"Lead on MacDuff."*

As they approached Dora, Betty stopped and started to laugh. *"Jings, is that what I think it is?"*

"Yes, it bloody is!" humped Dora.

Betty had texted Helen so she was waiting on her deck. *"God what have you come as?"* she laughed as she saw Betty's outfit.

Betty did not deign to answer, just tutted and threw a look over her shoulder.

WOMEN ON TOUR
ESSENTIAL SUPPLIES
MEETING OUR OWN NEEDS AT LAST

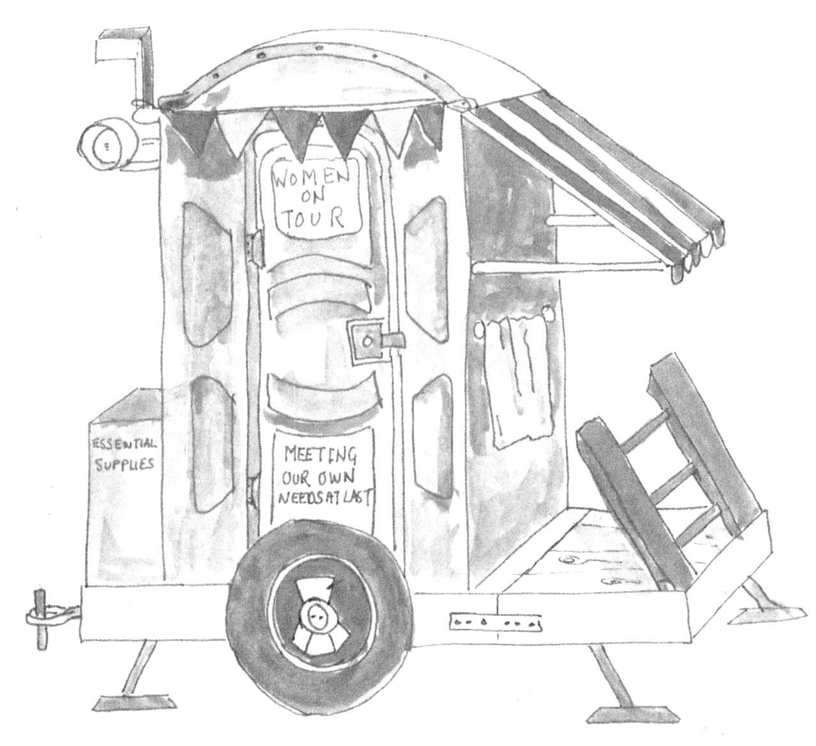

Fran slid open Dora's side door and Helen climbed up and dropped down onto Dora's back seat and sighed. She looked around her and then said: *"What the hell is that behind us?"*

"It's my shame," said Dora in a very resigned manner.

At Joni's house, there was no sign of her and the house looked deserted. Fran knocked and rang and finally got out her mobile phone.

"Yup," answered Joni.

"Are you ready, we are all here, you got the text?"

"Yeah, but I need help."

"Right open up and we will assess the damage." Fran gestured to the others and they crowded on Joni's step.

Eventually, the door opened and Joni appeared, the pain on her face told them all they needed to know. She was leaning forward on her crutches but her small suitcase was neatly stowed in the porch.

"Joni, are you really up for this?" asked Fran. *"You don't look great."*

"I'll be honest with you all; the thought of this trip is the only thing which has been keeping me going."

Joni started to move slowly forward, the rest parted and watched as she moved slowly down her front steps. She stopped and turned to face them all.

"Oh, I feel better already, what's that? Is that the facilities?" Joni laughed.

"She'll not be laughing when she tries to get into Dora," whispered Betty to Helen.

As they approached Dora Fran slid open the door and reached under the back seat and pulled out a ramp. *"There you go, all set."*

"I should be able to get in but that big box is in the way," said Joni.

"You mean the magic box?" said Fran.

"You know I never knew that was real," answered Joni.

"Oh yes it is very real and the contents are going to shape the next few days," said Dora.

"It's finally glowing," said Fran, *"let's open it."* She reached forward and slowly opened the box.

"Hit me with it," called Dora.

"Ok, there is a huge first aid kit, a pair of rowlocks wrapped up in survival blankets and a closed cardboard box."

The four old friends stood and stared into the magic box.

"This all looks a bit scary," stated Betty.

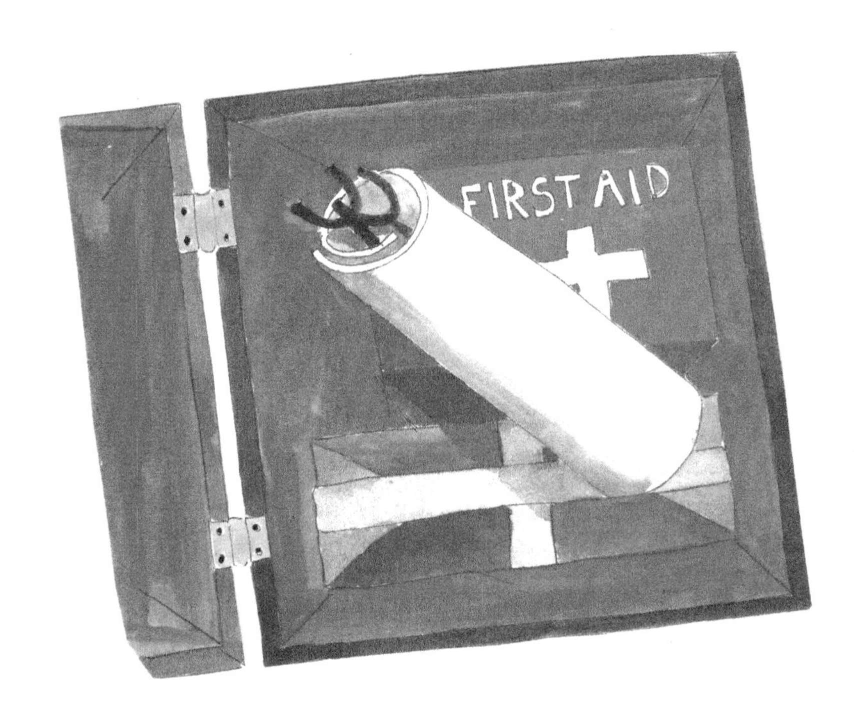

"Looks like we are going to be dealing with a major incident," laughed Joni, *"or perhaps it is just to meet my medical needs."*

"You know, there is never any point in trying to work out what's going to happen," stated Dora authoritatively, *"you just get in, we drive off and the adventure unfolds."*

"Well you know me," said Helen, *"I just go with the flow."*

The countryside flew past.

"How do you know where you are going Dora?" asked Joni, as she arranged her crutches, stretched out her legs and winced in pain.

"I don't know where I'm going," said Dora caustically. *"I'm a van."*

The mellow tones of Joni Mitchell's 'Court and Spark album' filled the van and for a time the women were quiet, each remembering times when they had been together in the past, things they had done and people they had known.

They drove along Loch Lomond, down Loch Long, its finger-shaped length disappearing into the distance and finally, they reached the head of Loch Fyne.

"Lunch stop," called Fran as she pulled into a lay-by at the top of the loch. Betty had fallen asleep and cricked her neck. She collapsed into one of the deck chairs which Fran had put out.

"Oh my god, I haven't even slept in the van yet and I am crooked," she moaned. Her neck was bent at an alarming angle and every time she tried to straighten it she gave a yelp.

"Well at least you can get out," moaned Joni as she stood, balanced precariously, looking nervously down at the ground which seemed a long way away.

"Come on Helen, let's help her down."

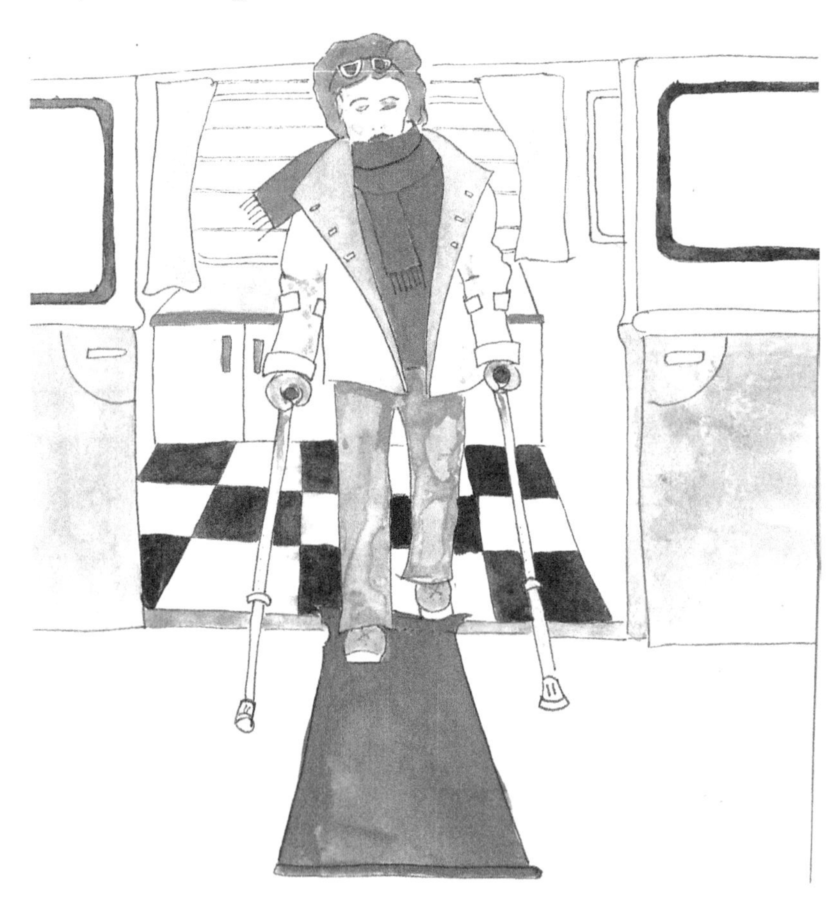

Fran located the ramp and with her arms around her friends' necks, Helen made her ungainly way down the ramp.

"Now I need to use the facility," she laughed.

Fran helped her round to the back of the trailer and pulled dramatically at a tarpaulin to reveal a complicated contraption. She raised a pole which resembled a mast and untangled a lot of ropes and a thing which looked like a sling.

"Right, sit on and we'll winch you up."

"WHIT?" screeched Joni.

"My god, you are joking!" Betty appeared and appraised the scene with her head still at its jaunty angle.

Just as Fran was lining Joni up with the canvas sling seat, Betty took out her phone and snapped a photo.

"You toad!" shouted Joni.

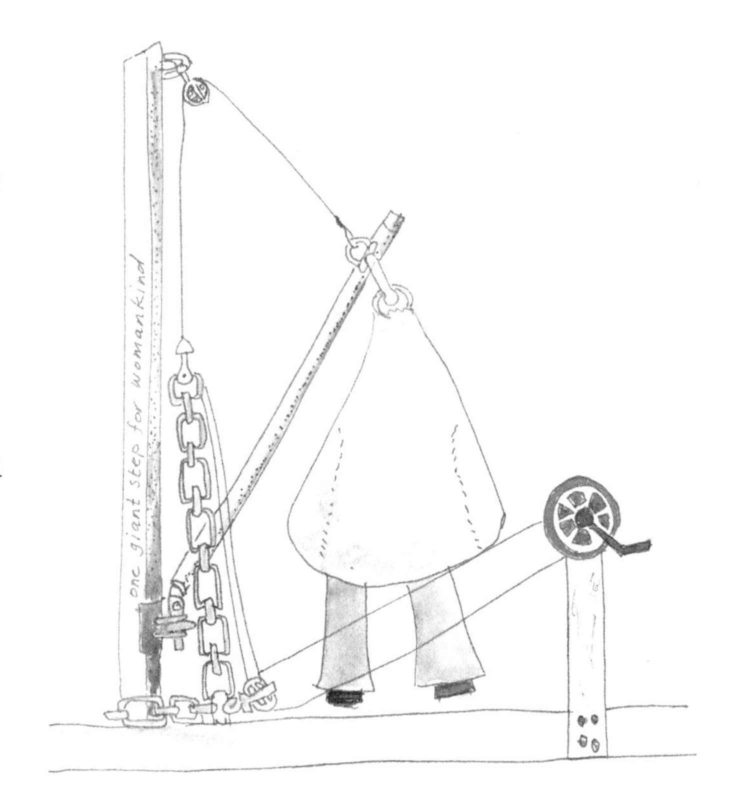

At that point, a quad bike carrying an elderly farmer and his very young collie drew up. The collie threw itself off the bike and started to jump up at Joni and bark wildly.

"Zayn, come here, Zayn."

The collie jumped back onto the bike, but the farmer remained seated, watching as Fran started to wind the wheel on the derrick and Joni started to swing and turn as she slowly rose into the air. The farmer stilled his collie and burst out laughing. *"Jings, criven's that's rare, that is rare."*

"Well, it's rare to find a man of your age who is a One Direction fan – and my hip will get better so..." Joni's response dried up.

"Aye well, that's grandchildren for you," stated the farmer. *"I don't even know who he is. When your hip is better I will make you an offer for yon contraption, it wid be brilliant for getting old sheep up onto the truck when they are off to the knackers yard."*

With that, he revved his engine and disappeared down a farm track.

"Fran, you might think you have thought this through but, jings, just look at me. And I've got to get down yet."

"Aye, well, is it an adventure? Did anybody die?" asked Fran.

"Not yet, but come on!"

"Well, the other facilities are just over there." Fran pointed at a tree.

"Ok, point taken."

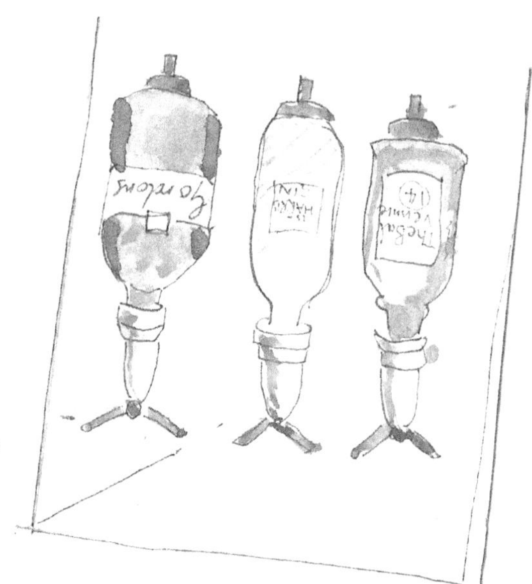

Fran opened a picnic hamper and laid out a beautiful lunch.

"What is in the 'emergency supplies' box Fran?" asked Hellen pointing to the trailer.

Fran reached over to reveal a set of optics, a set of glasses and a coolbox.

"Wey hey, now we're talking," laughed Betty as she tried to straighten her neck.

Following their lunch, Betty and Joni chose to have an afternoon nap while Fran and Helen set off for a walk along the shore. They chatted and poked around for driftwood and shells when Fran spotted a rowing boat drifting out, away from the shore on the tide.

"Oh dear someone didn't tie up their boat properly," she said as they watched as the boat drifted.

Fran was thinking about the rowlocks in the magic box but could see no need for them. They sat together as the boat drifted, the sun disappeared behind some dark clouds and it started to rain.

"Right back to Dora, we'll have to help Joni in out of this rain."

Fran stood reached to pull Helen up and turned away from the loch. Just then they heard a faint cry.

"There is someone in the boat, listen."

As they watched a dogs head appear and then the head of what was obviously a child. They could quite clearly hear crying.

"I'm going to swim out to the boat," said Helen. *"If I go round the loch a bit and get closer it's not a long swim."*

"Are you sure?"

"I go to the over 50's swim every Wednesday at our local pool, I'm sure," said Helen in a very determined voice.

"But, it'll be bloody freezing," stated Fran.

"Not for nothing all this blubber then?" laughed Helen grabbing the mass of her stomach and jiggling it.

"Right ok, but wait 'til I run to Dora and get the rowlocks and towels."

Fran left Helen to make her way around the loch as she jogged on her mission and to alert the others. Betty followed her back carrying the rowlocks and survival blankets, Fran carried towels while Joni was boiling kettles and phoning the emergency services.

"Helen, we don't think you should go in. Joni is phoning 999 and nobody is in real danger," stated Betty firmly.

"That child looked really young and it is getting cold," Helen said in a very determined voice.

At that point, Fran remembered that Helen had had an older brother who had died in a drowning accident. Then, as they watched in horror the child stood up, the boat wobbled dramatically and the child fell in.

"Take these!" Fran handed the rowlocks to Helen and she stuffed them down her pants as she ran into the water and threw herself head first into the dark cold loch.

Betty and Fran shouted to the child to encourage it to stay afloat. Helen streaked through the water and soon reached the child and hefted it onto the dinghy. She dragged herself onto the side of the boat but they could see that she was really struggling to climb in. Suddenly, she seemed to throw her bulk forward and all but disappeared into the boat only her feet waggling about in the air remained.

"Blimey, that was impressive," mouthed Betty.

Soon Helen had inserted the rowlocks and was rowing confidently back to shore.

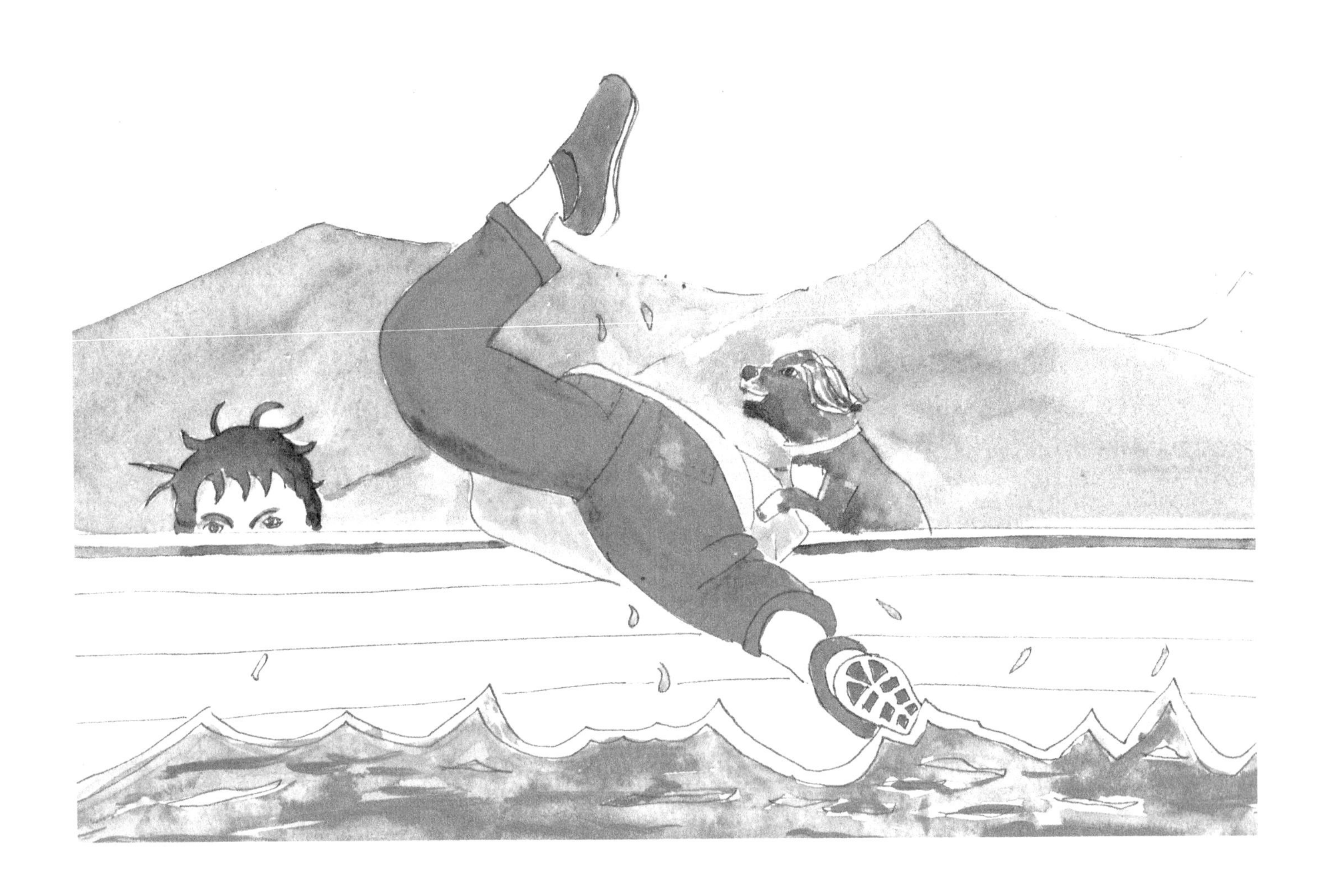

They could hear a siren, and, watched as the patrol car screamed around the bend and pulled off the road.

"We have been looking for wee Neil for hours, the wee devil. Nobody thought to see if he had taken the boat."

The policeman lifted the sobbing, freezing child from the boat and wrapped him in the emergency blanket.

"You seem to be very well prepared ladies, good job."

He turned away from them and spoke into his radio: *"Yes, he's safe, some old women have pulled him out. I'll bring him now. The situation is all under control."*

The man, boy and dog disappeared into the car which drove off swiftly down the lochside.

Back in Dora, Helen starting rooting in her bag for dry clothes. She tutted, *"I can't find my reiki pants."*

*"Ha, your **what**?"* laughed Fran.

Helen fixed Fran with a steely glare – *"My reiki pants, I feel the need for some healing and they will be the very dab."*

"Reiki pants," guffawed Joni, *"perhaps they can help my hip to heal, it is the right location."*

"Here!" Helen waved a jazzy pair of knickers in the air.

"What makes them Reiki Pants?" asked Betty.

"Well, the Reiki healer hovers their hands over them and...don't look at me like that Betty," warned Helen.

"Did you get them off that website where you can get the paw readings?"

"I've got a reiki basque you know," stated Fran in a deadpan voice.

"Ha, I need one of those," said Joni. *"For that..."* and she burst into song, *"...sexual healing."*

Three women burst out laughing and one looked angry.

"Right!" said Helen firmly. *"There are many ways of getting through the menopause and this is mine so... SHUT-UP!"*

There was an awkward silence and then, the diplomat as ever, Fran tried to clear the air.

"Today I forgot we were ladies of a certain age, even though that young man referred to us as 'old'. You know at my age, most of the time I feel invisible, but that felt great."

"Yes," added Helen. *"Today, I was bloody cold, but great. I felt capable and energised and alive."* Helen climbed into her pyjamas and sleeping bag to warm up and took a long pull of her drink. *"Sláinte, ladies. Here's to the next adventure. OH GOD!"*

"What's wrong?" asked Joni.

"Get me out of this sleeping bag; I am burning up, good god!"

"The next great adventure is getting us all into bed, we will just stay here, we're all set, aren't we Joni?"

"No comment."

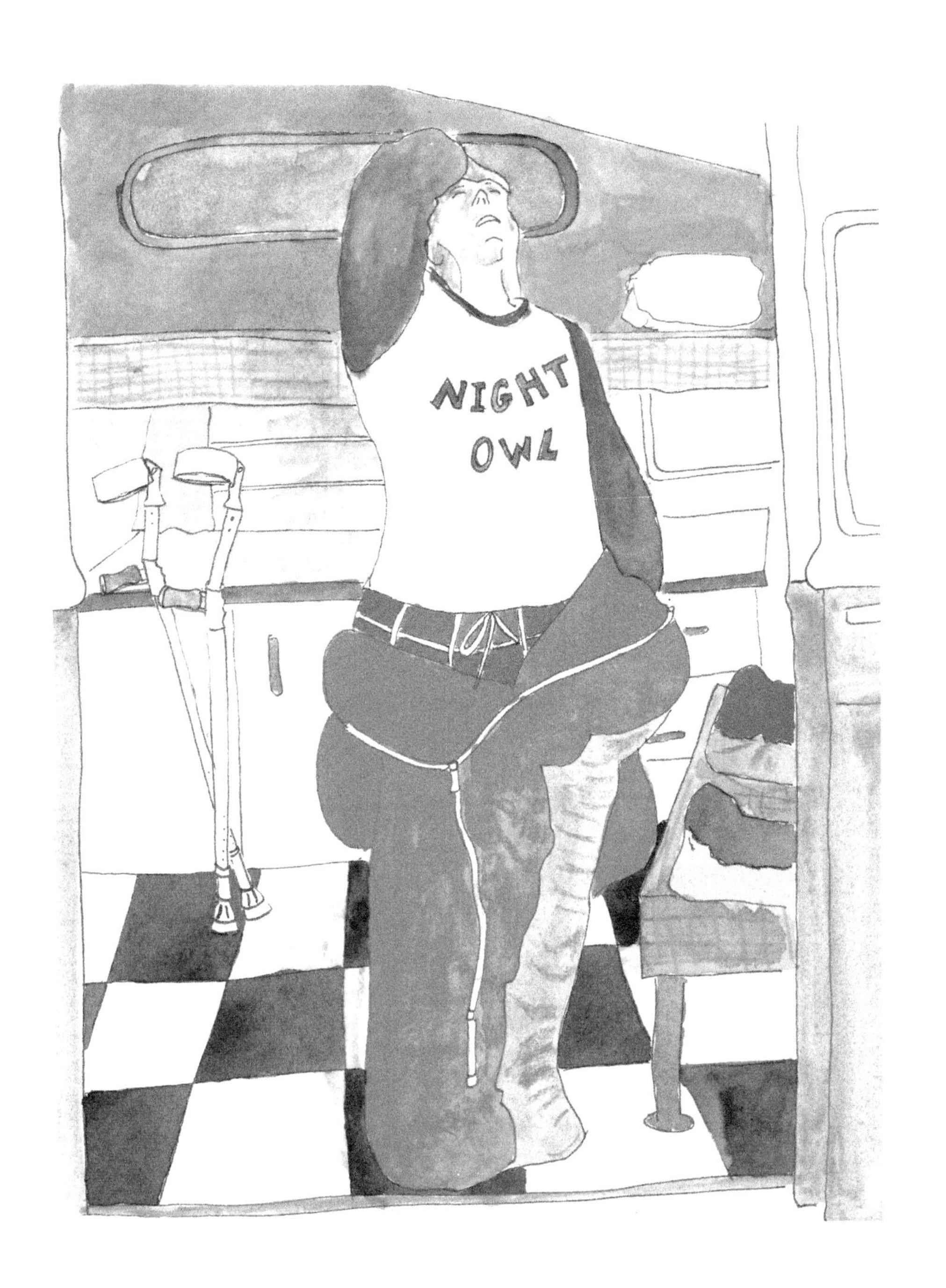
NIGHT
OWL

The dawn chorus started at four thirty and by five the four friends were fidgeting and restless.

"Anybody cold last night?" asked Fran from her precarious position in her upper bunk cot.

"Ha, cold, some chance," laughed Betty.

"You know once I got out of my bed at three o'clock in the morning to look up what caused these bloody flushes."

"And?" asked Helen.

"It is to do with the oestrogen leaving the body as it is one of the hormones which helps to regulate temperature in the brain, and that's not the worst thing," Betty paused for dramatic effect, *"the worst thing is... that the whole carry on can last for fifteen years."*

There was silence as three brains remembered almost forgotten arithmetic skills.

"Bloody ***age****strogen!"* moaned Helen. *"Every old lady I have ever met has said, 'if I could give you one bit of advice, dear, it is – don't get old.' Good advice indeed."*

"You know," said Dora, *"it really makes me laugh when you lot talk about being old. I am forty-three and that is one hundred and twenty-nine in van years."*

"Yes," countered Fran. *"But you don't have to feel old. We do live in a society which seems to be all about the youff, but we can buck the trend by getting out there and living."*

"Yes," added Dora, *"just keep your paintwork shiny and your engine fettled and keep on going."*

"Well, I don't know how I am going to get down from here," laughed Helen from the other upper bunk cot, *"but as soon as I work it out I am with you. Fran can you crack a window, it's a bit warm?"*

Fran let herself slide off her sleeping cot onto the floor and reached across to open the driver's window. She spotted a man jogging slowly towards them. She could hear he was singing. As he passed the bus, the four women convulsed into hysterics as his dulcet tones could be heard singing at the top of his voice: *"Tell me when will you be mine? Quando, quando quando, quando."*

"That's how you do it!" said Fran as she helped Helen lower herself down and reached for the kettle.

"Quando, quando, quando, quando," sang the women as they tidied away the night and got set for the day.

It was a slightly overcast Saturday as Dora puttered gently down Loch Fyne, through Inverary, and onto Lochgilphead. Just outside Lochgilphead Fran pulled the van into the carpark of the High School as there was a shinty match taking place between Kilmory and Oban Camanachd youth teams. There was a large crowd watching and much cheering and encouragement from the parents. Each of the friends made themselves comfortable on deck chairs with warm rugs. The match provided a great deal of entertainment. The watching crowd had brought an interesting range of shelters to keep out the cold wind – large umbrellas, beach tents, and even windbreaks.

Kilmory had just equaled the score at two-all, when a large fishing umbrella with a very pointy end broke free from its guy line and started to career across the pitch, followed by its distressed owner, who was screaming and shouting in panic. It hit two players on the head, felling them, it appeared to pierce the boot of the Buckshee forward, gained speed and headed towards the women.

Joni looked alarmed and then looked behind her as she was aware that three little girls were playing quietly in the grass while their elder siblings played shinty. With the exception of Joni, the women stood up and moved to the side.

"Joni, move!" shouted Fran.

But Joni held her own as the umbrella headed straight for her.

The umbrella bucked and jumped. Just as it reached her, Joni swiped at it with her crutch and hoisted it into the air where it was caught by the wind and thrown across the road and into the Loch. After the screaming and shouting there was silence and then a spontaneous round of applause and effuse thanks from the parents of the little girls.

Fran became aware of Dora peeping and flashing her lights.

"I am just going to collect the first aid kit. Betty, Helen can you gather the wounded?"

As the umbrella drifting out into the loch with the tide, Betty and Helen dealt with the various cuts and scratches. Fran eased the boot off the foot of the Buckshee forward. He was ashen and blood seeped from a nasty gash. She got him to sit down and applied pressure. Joni hobbled over on her crutches and covered him with her blanket. The home team coach had phoned 999 and soon sirens could be heard. A squad car and an ambulance drew up. The young policeman who had attended the boat incident the day before appeared at Fran's side.

"You again!" they both said at the same time.

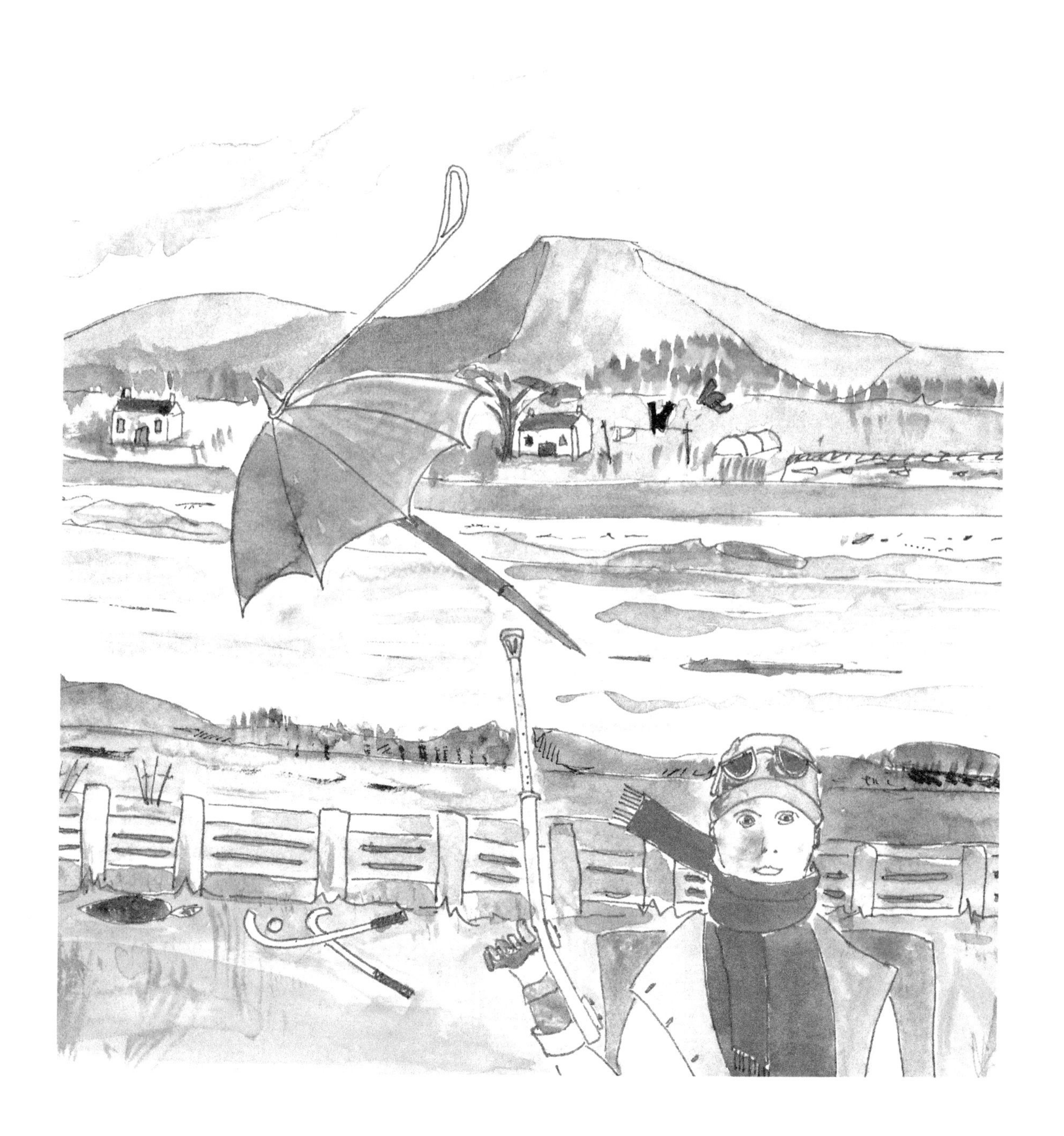

"Yes," laughed Fran, *"us again, us old women dealing with the situation and bringing calm."*

"Ah right, well the ambulance is here now," he said, not sure how to respond.

Finally, the scene cleared and the women climbed back into Dora. Just as Dora fired into life, the team coach ran over and knocked on the window.

"We are having a ceilidh tonight in the school hall, please come as our guests, we are very grateful for your help today."

He indicated behind him. *"Just here, starts at seven, please come."* He smiled and waved as Dora made her way sedately down the school drive.

"Well ladies, think we raised our game today. You know Fran, this really is becoming an adventure. I just feel great, we must make this at least an annual event." Betty reached across and patted her friend on the arm.

Fran's heart sang. She had missed her trips in Dora since the kids had grown up and this was going better than she could ever have expected.

"Thank-you Betty that is exactly how I feel."

"Quando, quando, quando, quando," sang Joni.

"We have one more problem to solve," stated Helen, *"we have nothing to wear tonight."*

"Look, look!" shouted Joni. *"The magic box, it's glowing again."*

Fran pulled into the side of the road and they slowly opened the box. The previously tightly shut cardboard box was open. Fran reached in and pulled out four black dresses each bearing a blue sunflower and a label with their names; Fran passed the dresses to the excited women. As the last dress was given out the magic box disappeared. The women held the dresses up and exclaimed.

"This is magic," stated Betty.

"Of course it is," answered Dora.

"You see the magic is always there, you just have to let it in."

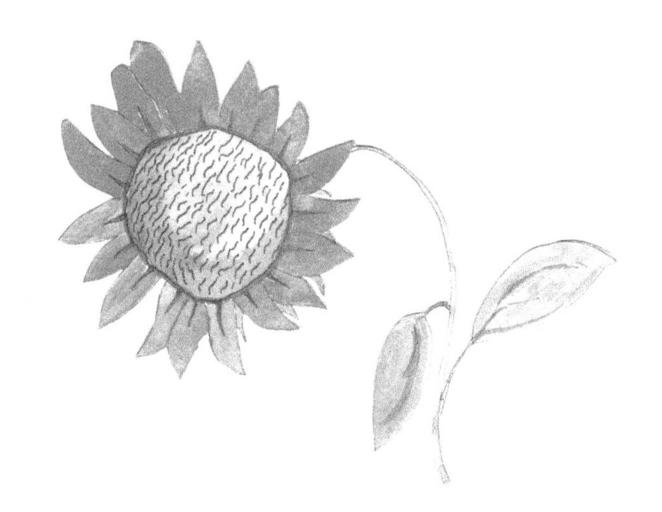

Later Dora again drove into the High School car park. The women helped Joni down and they swept up to the open doors.

As they entered the school hall, dressed in its tartan banners with the Argyll ceilidh band playing a lively reel, the women could feel all eyes were upon them.

"Look," shouted a loud voice, *"it's the calendar girls!"*

Fran turned to her friends and said: *"No, we're ...*

... Dora's girls."

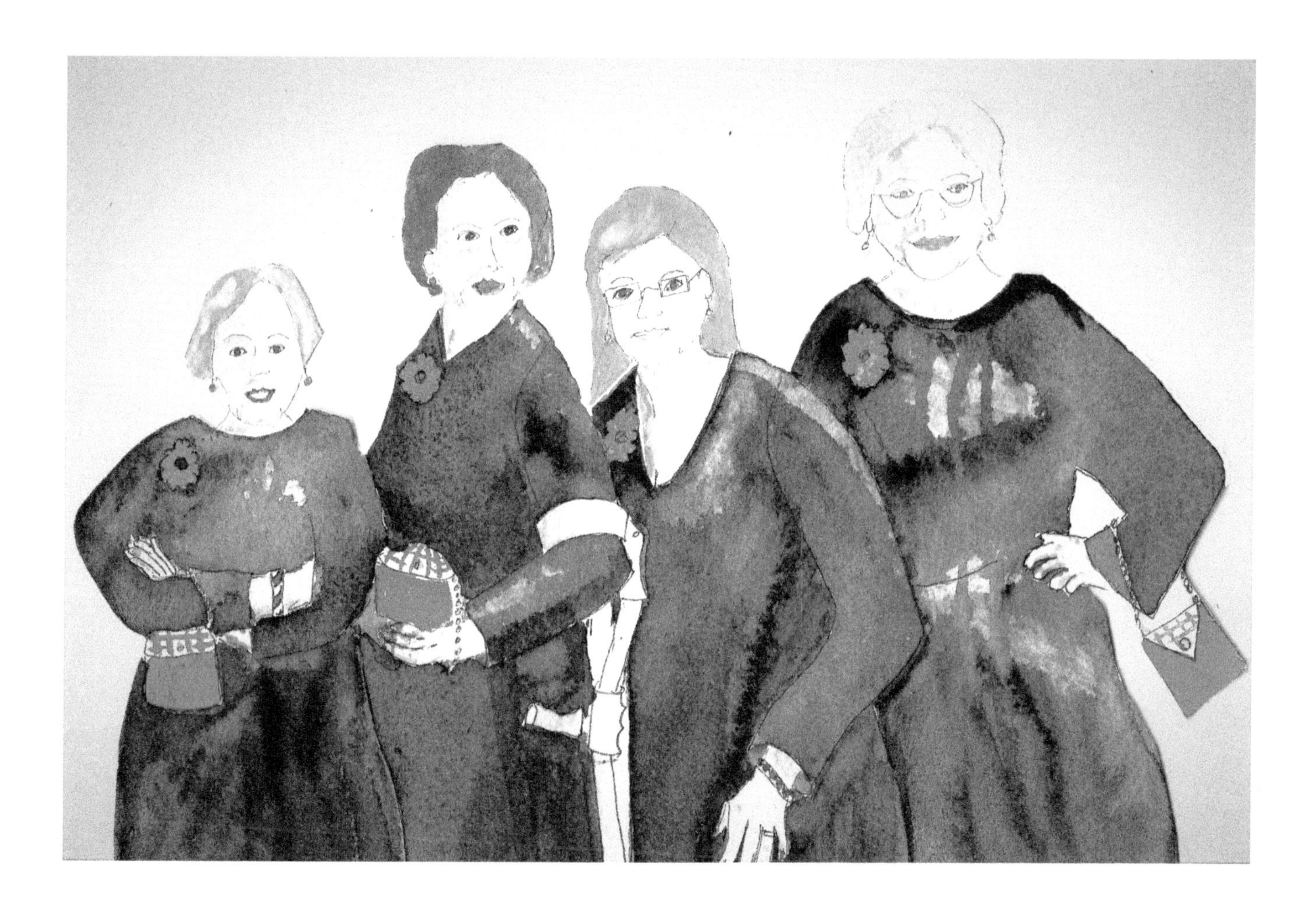

About the Author

Frances Herbert is a retired teacher who loves the West of Scotland and Volkswagen Camper Vans of a certain age.

Also by Frances Herbert (for the grandchildren!):

Fran's Van and the Magic Box

Fran's Van and the Naughty Border Terrier

Fran's Van and the Beach of the Winds

Fran's Van and the Arran Adventure

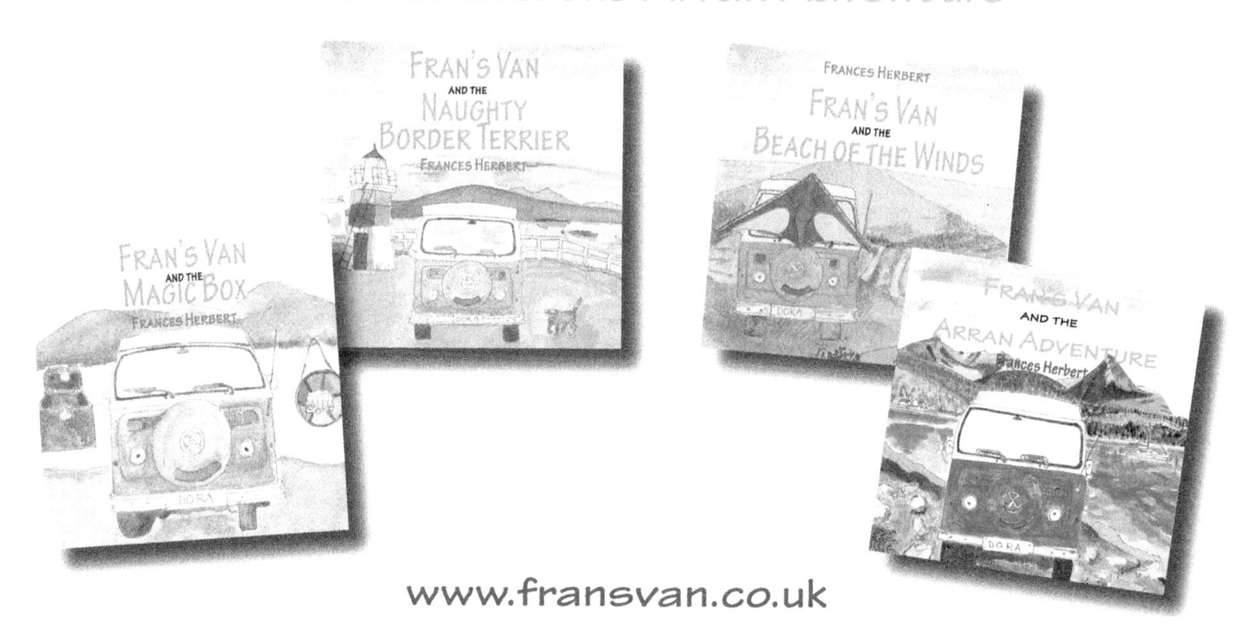

www.fransvan.co.uk

Lightning Source UK Ltd.
Milton Keynes UK
UKOW07f1125071217
314047UK00005B/68/P

9 781782 225614